Gabriel N.

A HEALTHY GUIDE
To
Eating

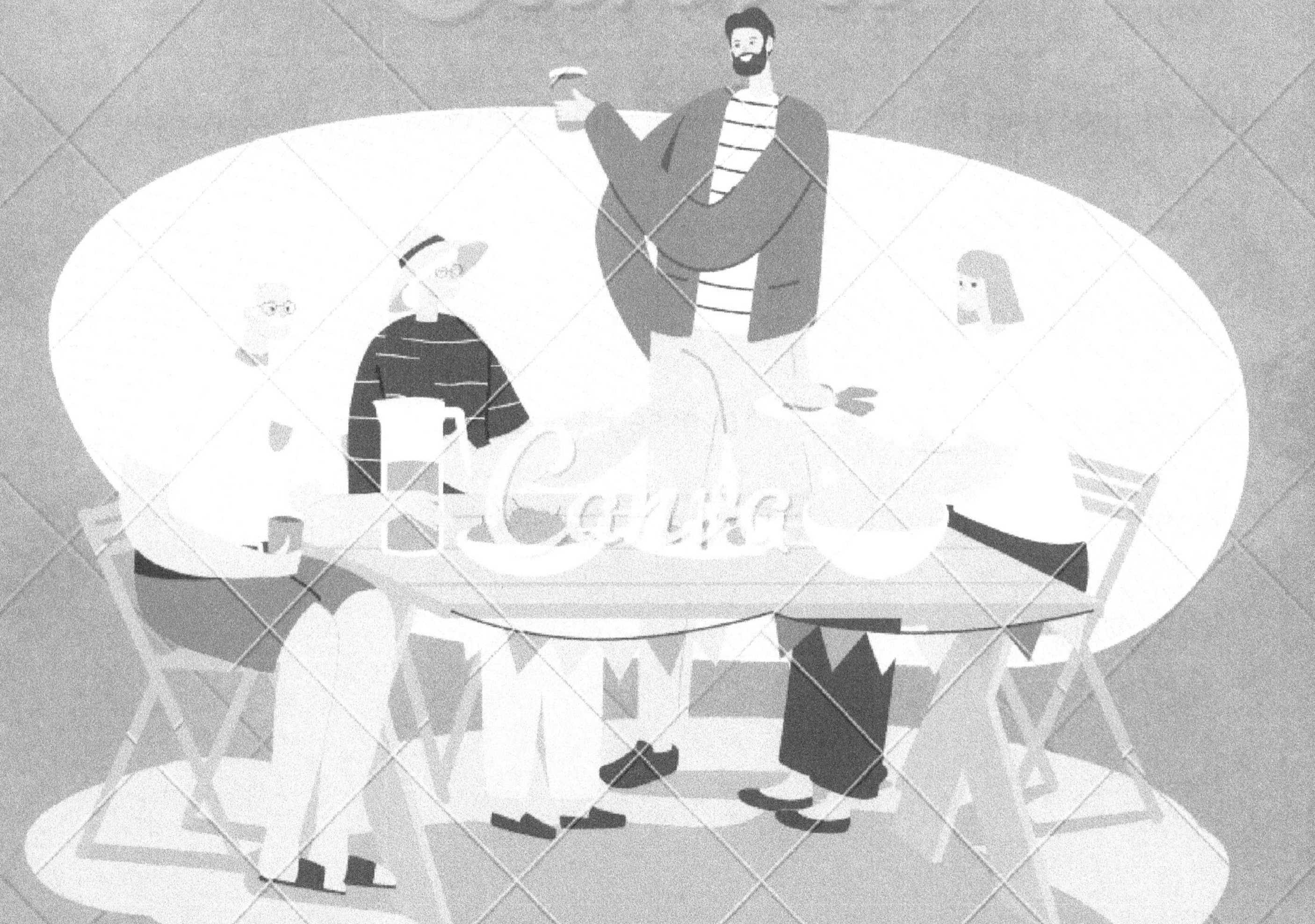

CONTENTS

INTRODUCTION

For some reason, one of the hardest things for a human to do is to eat right. Whether that is because we have limited access to resources in all areas or if it is because we simply have too much access to unhealthy food, there are many reasons that eating healthy is a challenge.

Sure, we can eat just about anything and it will sustain us. We will manage to move from one moment to the next and be able to call ourselves healthy. But is it healthy to subsist on a diet of processed foods and sugary drinks? Just because we are alive does not mean that we are healthy. And the older we get, the more our bad habits begin to catch up with us.

It is unbelievably important to form healthy eating habits early on in life, or at least, as early as possible to prevent any future issues from occurring. You do not want to wake up one day and realize that you have had a nutrient deficiency for years and it is causing complications that are almost impossible to rectify. All of us need to take more responsibility for what we put into our bodies, because if we don't, it can become extremely dangerous.

Of course, when we are older and we are able to look back on our mistakes, hindsight is 20/20. We realize that there were things that we could have done and probably should have done that we simply didn't do because we were either unconscious of the ill effects, or simply lazy. Just having the simple knowledge does not necessarily make then needs to do something health- conscious a reality.

For the most part, it takes us truly being exposed to the

suffering
that can occur because of bad health choices before we are
more
conscious of the way we treat our bodies and our health in general. When we aren't able to see the reality of the consequences to our actions, it can make them feel

very far away and difficult to relate to. We may even blow them off entirely. This can be a very debilitating place to find yourself in. Especially when you are already dealing from the side effects of poor eating and a lack of a healthy diet.

Everybody deserves a chance to become the greatest version of themselves possible, but if we are not even acknowledging the fact that unhealthy eating can take us right off course, even in the present moment, then we are ultimately waving goodbye to the best future possible.

But all of this can change. By reading this book, you are going to understand the importance of eating healthy and how food impacts our bodies and functions.

Without understanding exactly why our bodies react to food the way they do, it can sometimes be difficult to stay on track. But there are many ways that you can begin to understand why eating healthy foods is so important, and exactly how to begin on a healthy eating journey. Let's not waste any more time. We should begin eating healthy today!

CHAPTER 1: WHY EAT HEALTHY?

Healthy eating is important for a lot of reasons. Most of us are already aware of the increasing obesity epidemic in North America. This is particularly true of the United States in general. There is even a phrase for the way many Americans eat, and that is called the SAD diet.

SAD stands for standard American diet, and it refers to a diet low in vegetables, high in fat and sugar, and lacking in nutrition. Processed foods are definitely a part of the SAD diet. These are foods that are easily available and quick to consume and prepare but have long-lasting negative health effects.

If you do not want to find yourself obese, it is generally considered a good idea to avoid eating such processed foods and keep your focus on eating whole grains and fruits and vegetables and meat that has not been treated with hormones and other chemicals that can ultimately end up in your body and cause issues. Unfortunately, in North America, we are given a lot of options to slack off when it comes to preparing meals.

We have so many things readily available to us, and the amount of money that you have to spend to buy bad food is far less then it is to buy good food. It seems strange that it costs more money to buy organic than it does to buy foods that will ultimately cause health problems in the long run, but that is the rule of supply and demand.

Not only that, but processed foods are mass-produced and

make
a huge profit because of their convenience. That is why, in many ways, and obesity epidemic in North America is not particularly surprising. Nutrition is not number one on the list of companies that are attempting to cash in on people's laziness in the

kitchen.

However, there are many ways that eating healthy is important, and good reasons to avoid processed foods and the standard American diet. For example, if you do not want to be obese, you should definitely look into the rest of this book for ways to improve your diet and begin a healthier lifestyle.

Another reason to eat healthy is because you can make yourself prone to diseases by eating unhealthy foods and by staying on a standard American diet that is full of fat and sugar. Diabetes is something that can be developed because of poor eating and can
often times be treated with healthy eating.

When you realize the impact and importance of your future and making positive choices about these things, it can make you more primed toward healthy eating and less inclined to make choices that negatively impact you and your future.

To be truthful, many of us seem to consider the future bleak. We do not see reasons enough to change our habits because if we do not believe that we have anything good to look forward to, then it doesn't matter whether we make good choices or not. We do not see how we can actually pave our future to be in our best interests. Probably because we do not believe that we have any power over our lives.

If you can relate to this feeling, don't be alarmed. It is very common of the human experience. We are generally discouraged from taking control and utilizing our power from an early age, and sometimes stopped believing we have any authority over our lives because we are usually told what to do by other people.

As children, that makes sense. Children don't always know what is best for them. But it can encourage a very helpless type of mindset that causes us to have a hard time understanding that the consequences of our actions can truly begin to shape who we are and how we present ourselves to the world.

CHAPTER 2: UNDERSTANDING YOUR RELATIONSHIP WITH FOOD

Over the course of time, everybody begins to develop certain habits. We develop habits in all arenas of our lives. We develop hygiene habits, food habits, work habits, and all sorts of other types of habits. However, they are usually pretty oblivious to our habits until they

begin to affect us negatively. And even then, when we begin to understand that we are being poorly impacted by our habits, it can be very difficult to change them. Because that is what I have it is like.

A habit is something that we do almost unconsciously. We are programmed to follow these habits, and it takes a great amount of willpower to break free from the cycle.

Once you begin to understand that your relationship with food has everything to do with the habits that you have created and habits that you can continue to mold and cultivate, then it becomes far easier to change your mindset.

When you realize the impact and importance of your future and making positive choices about these things, it can make you more primed toward healthy eating and less inclined to make choices that negatively impact you and your future.

To be truthful, many of us seem to consider the future bleak. We do not see reasons enough to change our habits because if we do not believe that we have anything good to look forward to, then it doesn't matter whether we make good choices or not. We do not see how we can actually pave our future to be in our best interests. Probably because we do not believe that we have any power over our lives.

If you can relate to this feeling, don't be alarmed. It is very common of the human experience. We are generally discouraged from taking control and utilizing our power from an early age, and sometimes stopped believing we have any authority over our lives because we are usually told what to do by other people.

As children, that makes sense. Children don't always know what is best for them. But it can encourage a very helpless type of mindset that causes us to have a hard time understanding that the consequences of our actions can truly begin to shape who we are and how we present ourselves to the world.

journey. All of us can take steps every day toward becoming our best possible selves, and healthy eating is one great step in that direction. And it is a step we can take today!

you eat healthy sometimes or not. The negative effects will still be gripping your body and waiting to spring up on you when you least expect it.

In a way, unhealthy eating is a self-destructive pattern that a lot of us take part in. Whether this is because of poor self-esteem, or simply because we are unhappy with our situations and have no faith in the future, self-destructive eating patterns are dangerous. You have to look to yourself and truly value your life and your future before eating healthy will stick.

There are many ways that you can do this, and if possible, you may even want to consult a mental health professional for support. Sometimes, they can help us to see biases and

negative
patterns in our lives that we remain oblivious to. Once those are understood and accepted, then it can be that much easier to overcome them and take the steps that you need to take in order
to make positive choices.

Whether you seek out the help of a qualified professional or not, there are many things that you can do to change your mindset. As long as you understand that you are worthy of a healthy body and a positive future, then you will allow yourself to take the steps necessary to get there.

But if you do not feel good about yourself, it is going to be a lot harder. Overall, understanding yourself, your habits, your mental roadblocks, and your discipline, will help you in your journey. All of us can take steps every day toward becoming our best possible selves, and healthy eating is one great step in that direction. And it is a step we can take today!

CHAPTER 3: THE DANGERS OF DIET TRENDS

Diet trends are rampant in our society today, and almost all of them come with dangers attached to them. Unfortunately, most people who are desperate to make money often don't look at the long-term health consequences of their products. What they are truly concerned about is making money and doing something that will help them to capitalize off of a desperate desire that many people have to lose weight in a fast and easy way.

There is something that you are going to have to accept if diet trends are something that captivate your interest. The unfortunate fact of the matter is that there is no healthy way to lose weight fast and easily with no work and no healthy eating and no exercise. Losing weight is a good goal if you are obese or if you are lacking in fitness and you need extra mobility.

All of us have at times needed to start making better lifestyle choices, and that is something that we can do with food and healthy body movement as opposed to by trusting companies that want to exploit us in order to make money.

Some of the diet trends out there are exceptionally dangerous and have dire health consequences both long-term and short-term. Many of them rely on methods that cause us to starve ourselves and Robert body of essential nutrients. Sometimes, even dehydrating us.

These types of diet trends are extremely disgusting. They are taking advantage of people who want to be healthy but don't know how to go about it. They are taking advantage of people, often women in particular, who are crumbling under the pressures of unrealistic beauty standards and women who are told that to have any value, they must look a certain way.

That is absolutely untrue. Whether you weigh 100 pounds or

700

pounds, you have value. However, healthy eating is one of the only real ways that you are going to be able to kickstart your metabolism and provide your body with the nutrients that it needs to function on its highest possible capacity.

If you are robbing your body of the vitamins and minerals that it needs in order to thrive and trusting a diet trend to teach you how to lose weight and have value when all they really want is your money, then you are going to end up further behind the line then you were to start out with. The unfortunate truth about many diet trends is that they cause the body to go into starvation

mode.

This can wreck your metabolism and cause you to gain weight even faster in the future. Don't let yourself be exploited by the advertisements promising that you will lose weight in a fast and easy way. All of that will come with a price. Not only that, but there are health trends out there such as the hCG diet that can really screw up your body and your hormones.

The ironic thing about diet trends is that they often will make it harder for you to lose weight in the future because you are implementing unhealthy and difficult ways of maintaining your weight. If you want to be skinny, don't trust a pill on TV to make you skinny. Start cutting out unhealthy sugary and processed foods and replace them with healthy whole-grain wheat and organic fruits and vegetables that will not introduce chemicals into your body that will make it even harder for you to lose weight and that will ultimately mess up your body chemistry.

It may seem tempting to be able to lose weight quickly and not have to sacrifice the negative eating habits that you have developed over your lifetime, but it is not healthy. You are hurting yourself and priming your body for further health complications in the future if you are not careful about the way you attempt to lose weight. Make sure that you are doing everything in your power to make choices that you would want other people to make for themselves.

Do research before you let yourself be swayed by the snake oil salesman on TV. Look into these things because you are worth doing things the right way and you deserve a positive future and not one that is complicated by the side effects of a sales pitch that only wants your money and not your health.

CHAPTER 4: THE FOOD PYRAMID

Most of us have probably seen the food pyramid. Growing up, the food pyramid was often used as a guideline for us to provide us with an idea of how much food and what kind of food we should eat every day in order to maintain a healthy lifestyle.

Of course, there is always evidence to state that the food pyramid is flexible, but overall, if you are able to observe the food pyramid you will have a general idea of what is acceptable in a healthy and nutritious diet.

While this may sometimes be controversial, it is still good to have a basic food. Possibly one that you create yourself. A lot of people will say that it is no longer considered the most healthy thing to do to eat as many grains as the food pyramid may have suggested.

In fact, with recent outbreaks of celiac disease, a lot of people are touting a no grain lifestyle as the most healthy choice.

Rather than relying on the food pyramid for your basic guideline of what is healthy to eat, try to take into consideration your own personal experiences with food and go from there. Some people are healthier with a lot of grains, and some are not. Use your judgment here to the best of your ability so that you will be able to take steps in the right direction for your health.

The standard food pyramid recommends as follows:

• Rice, cereal, pasta, and bread, can be as many as 11 servings per day.

• For vegetables and fruits, you should have between three and five servings.

• As far as their eggs, you can have two or three servings every day, provided you are not allergic or lactose intolerant.

• When it comes to meet and beans, and other things like nuts and fish or poultry, it is recommended that you have two or three servings every day.

• Unsurprisingly, things such as sugar and fat and oil are the very tip of the. Because you should not have any of these things in excess. Rather, use them only as necessary in order to guarantee your healthiest possible lifestyle.

Again, this is only referencing the standard food pyramid. Depending on your own singular needs and dietary functions, you may need to modify this chart for yourself. But if you do not have any specific requirements, this is the standard for the food pyramid that can be utilized to your greatest possible advantage in creating a healthier lifestyle.

CHAPTER 5: HOW FOOD CAN BE YOUR MEDICINE

The same way that not eating healthy can make you sick, eating healthy foods can often times cure you of illness and provide you with relief when you are suffering.

It can also act as a preventative measure to take against illness. In fact, there is an entire method of healing around India for thousands of years called Aryuveda.

This ancient healing style is utilized in order to treat any illness simply by changing your diet. Food is literally the medicine that has helped to keep the people of India alive for centuries. And it can still be applicable today.

In fact, many remedies are simply healthy foods that have anti-inflammatory properties and the ability to nourish your body from the inside out. Everything from infection to cancer has been known to be impacted by healthy eating choices.

And with this ancient healing art, that has never been more apparent.

Of course a lot of modern technology will frown upon these methods because they have not been scientifically investigated, but a lot of it has been tried and true for thousands of years and will continue to impact the body.

Whether you believe in the ancient healing art or not, the fact remains that food can ultimately determine whether or not you are susceptible to illness. If you eat well, your body will be stronger and it will be able to fight off illness and infection far easier than it would if you find yourself malnourished on standard American diet.

Without the proper vitamins and minerals in your body, it can be almost impossible to fight off the negative effects of illness. Sometimes, it can even cause illness. If you are eating

unhealthy
unprocessed foods, certain types of these foods can actually lead
to illnesses and make you more susceptible to certain types of cancer as well.

Although cancer is still being researched and has not fully been understood by the scientific community well enough to actually cure it, there are many instances of people who were able to live long and healthy lives simply by changing the way they need. Healthy eating can help in decreasing the symptoms of many difficult and impossible to cure diseases, such as multiple sclerosis.

As long as you are making sure that everything that you put into your body is nourishing and is providing your organs and cells with all of the fuel and resources that they need in order to keep your body strong, they will continue to do that. And they will do it to the best of their ability.

However, if you are actively sabotaging your body, they will not be able to put up the same fight as they would if they were receiving adequate nutrition. That is why it is so important for you to take heed of the way you are nourishing your body. If you are not making active and conscientious choices about the food that you eat, you could be setting yourself up for failure in ways that you may live to regret.

CHAPTER 6: THE HEALTH BENEFITS OF EATING VEGETABLES

Vegetables are one of the most under-sung foods in existence, especially when it comes to the standard American diet. Most people don't realize just how important it is to provide the body with the vitamins and minerals that vegetables and vegetables alone can provide. Sometimes, people will look into vegetables as a way of improving their beauty, but when it comes to improving their health, they become somewhat disinterested.

However, now that you are here and reading this book, it is safe to assume that you are willing and able to take into consideration why it is important to eat vegetables. Here are some of the best reasons to provide yourself with vegetables daily as a part of your diet.

First of all, the body needs fiber in order to get rid of excess waste. Without a way to find the waste together and eliminated, it stays stuck in the body and can contribute to weight gain and other potential complications.

Fiber is extremely important for other reasons as well. It can help you to prevent your blood cholesterol from raising and can even prevent heart disease, or at least lower the chances of suffering from it.

Folic acid it is also present in vegetables, and when you are providing your body with this substance, it can generate the production of your red blood cells. This can be very important in helping you to prevent anemia from occurring, and can be very beneficial to women in particular, who have a tendency to need this substance during pregnancy and menstruation.

Vegetables are also naturally high in many vitamins, such as a and C, which are helpful in fighting infection and keeping the body healthy. It can help you to speed up the healing process and to absorb iron, which is another way of helping to combat and prevent anemia from occurring. Vitamins are high in potassium and this is very useful because it prevents the body from succumbing to high blood pressure.

Vegetables have been proven to reduce the risk of strokes and other heart related complications. They can prevent kidney stones from developing and prevent the disintegration of bone matter. Filling yourself up on vegetables is a good way to help you to manage type II diabetes and obesity.

Not only that, but it can help you to stay strong in a fight against cancer and in cancer prevention. Perhaps one of the most to stop acne in its tracks by keeping your body free of waste products that come out through your pores and hydrating your skin. Fruit is excellent for helping the body to stay hydrated because of its high water content, and you will quickly begin to see the benefits and that aspect.

Not only that, but fruit is particularly helpful for digestion. Because of the high fiber content, it helps to bind waste and help the body to eliminate things that might otherwise cause issues. Because of this, fruit and vegetables can also aid in weight loss. Rather than allowing waste to be broken down and stored as fat, the body eliminates it before it has the chance.

Fruit is another great way to help you to fight and prevent disease, even cancer. Some fruits, such as apples, help to keep asthma at bay. Others, can significantly lower cholesterol levels.

Grapes have been known to be used in the combat of cancer as well, particularly the red skinned grapes. They are also helpful in fighting eye issues and kidney problems. If you suffer from infection, berries are especially helpful. They are high in antioxidants.

Just make sure that you are eating fruits and vegetables that are not treated with commercial pesticides, as they can absorb these chemicals and actually complicate weight loss and cause issues in the body.

You can even eat dry fruits as a way of substituting unhealthy and sugary snacks and providing your body with a sweet snack that will pack quite a nutritional punch. Just be conscientious of the sugar levels in dried fruits, because sometimes when they are commercially sold, added sugars make what could be a healthy treat into something that may ultimately help you to pack on the pounds.

However, when you are eating fruit in a healthy way and on a regular basis, fruit can help to aid you in weight loss. As long as you are not over eating things that are high in sugar, the fibers and water content of fruit will help your body feel full and your cells and organs nourished. The fibers and water content will help you to eliminate issues that are contributing to obesity, and overall you will feel an immense shift in your energy levels.

You can utilize this energy to exercise and work harder toward a healthy lifestyle. This can be especially effective if you are replacing sugary junk foods with healthier fruit alternatives as you continue to transition on your journey toward better health and well-being.

CHAPTER 8: THE BEST MEAT TO EAT FOR HEALTHY LIVING

Meat is generally considered one of the primary staple foods in an email, but it may be surprising to find that there are actually some meats that are healthier than others. Of course, we know the difference between red meats and white meats. Red meats are more often linked to health problems and coronary issues, while white meats are considered leaner and healthier overall.

What some people may be surprised to find is that there are other issues that make meats unhealthy. Issues such as the things that they are fed while the animals are still alive and antibiotics and hormones that may be injected into them to make them grow faster or produce more milk, at least in the case of cows.

These types of hormones ultimately enter the meat that we consume and can cause problems in our own bodies. If we are not conscientious of the choices that we make when we are choosing our foods, they can ultimately come to contribute to poor health in the future, including but not limited to cancers and hormone changes that can be quite debilitating.

However, if you are confident that you are receiving your meat from sources that are healthy and do not feed animals in excess of steroids and antibiotics, then you are already ahead of the game. If not, try to do some research about local places where you can receive meat that is untainted by some dangerous industry standards.

That being said, even considering the healthy meat options, there are certain meats that are healthier than others. One of the healthiest meats that you can eat, especially if you are hoping to lose weight, is fish. Fish is lean and packed with nutrients. However, you have to be careful about the source of your fish.

Some fish is raised in unhealthy conditions, while other fish may come from areas that could be contaminated with mercury. This is why it is frowned upon for pregnant women to eat fish or shellfish.

But if you find a healthy source of fish, this can be very

beneficial
for your body. Fish is high in omega-3 fatty acids, which helps brain function and your memory. Overall, Omega threes are highly coveted and the body needs them in order to function at its highest possible potential, especially when it comes to intellectual matters.

Chicken that has been raised in a good environment is another great option. Chicken is high in protein. In fact, it is the highest in protein of any other meat. They are usually raised in good conditions, or at least fed foods that will not cause the human body issues the same way a lot of beef can.

However, if you are eating grass that beef from a trustworthy supplier, that can also be a great option as well. If you are going to eat organic chicken, there are generally less likelihoods of these animals being raised with dangerous carcinogens.

Chickens that have been conventionally grown are usually fed foods that increase the rate that they grow, which can lead to serious health problems for the chickens themselves and for the humans that consume them. They are also given a large supply of antidepressants and painkillers, sometimes, even arsenic and caffeine.

It is dangerous to consume a lot of conventionally grown meat, but if you are able to find a good supplier, then you definitely should do so.

Turkey is another great meat, because it is high in selenium.

This
is something that is great for the body, especially because it can help to eliminate free radicals and other toxic substances.

Again though, you want to try to make sure that you are receiving your meat from trustworthy sources, because it is standard for conventionally grown chicken and turkey is to be treated similarly and fed dangerous chemicals that unnaturally increase their rate of growth and ultimately contaminate human bodies with those chemicals.

Eating meat overall can be very beneficial for the body, as long as you are not eating meat that comes from dangerous and conventionally grown methods. The chemicals that these animals are often subject to our exceptionally dangerous, both to the animals themselves and to the humans who consume them. If you want to eat healthy and lose weight, it is better to avoid any chemicals that may end up staying stuck in your body and preventing weight loss from occurring.

Even if you are not hoping to lose weight, eating healthy

includes
avoiding anything that could be dangerous to the body, such as the hormones and chemicals that are disruptive to our sensitive systems. Fortunately, there are many sources for healthy meats, whether you want to indulge in chicken, beef, or even lamb. There are ways that you can get healthy, ethically raised me to satisfy any cravings you may have.

CHAPTER 9: THE DANGERS OF PROCESSED FOODS

It does not come as a surprise to anybody that processed foods are dangerous. What does come as a surprise however is that they are still allowed out on the shelves, despite the havoc that they wreak on our bodies and minds. Eating unhealthy food isn't just a personal choice to some people.

Sometimes, because of the way the economy works, people in poverty are forced to turn to processed foods because they are a cheap and easy way to feed large families on a low budget.

The hard thing about that is that these foods ultimately cause medical problems down the line that cost even more money than it would take to feed a large family healthy, sustainable options. Ultimately, it seems that people with little money are suffering either way.

Even if you don't have to feed a family on a budget, processed foods are simply unhealthy. Part of what makes them so addicting is their high fat and sugar content.

They are often boxed meals that include pastas and an exceptional amount of sugar. Excessive sugar is dangerous in general, but especially to people who are prone to developing type II diabetes. If you consume sugar and high amounts, you are ultimately going to overload your body and not only will you become obese, more than likely, but you also develop health issues.

Sugar can help speed along the process of diabetes because of the fact that it causes insulin resistance to occur which ultimately
makes it difficult, if not impossible, to control your blood sugar levels.

If you eat foods like this excessively, such as for every meal, or

at
least every day, there is bound to be a negative consequence. Consuming that high amount of fat and sugar on a consistent basis can lead to not only diabetes and obesity, which are commonly known, but also heart disease and even cancer. This is exceptionally dangerous, and if possible, processed foods should be avoided at all costs.

Another danger of eating processed foods is that not only are they addicting, but they are highly artificial. Most of the ingredients in those foods are not nourishing the body. Rather, they are leading us to feel full while depriving our bodies of the essential nutrients that are required in healthy functioning.

When we are eating a diet that is bland and not nourishing, we are ultimately allowing ourselves to be dumbed down. We are not thinking properly, we are not moving properly, and we are not functioning at her highest possible potential. All of these things are highly damaging and can lead to poor coordination and even depression.

On some level, we all know that processed foods are not as healthy as the types of foods we should be consuming on a regular basis. Our bodies know it, even if our minds are not aware. And we suffer for it. We have stress about it.

When we indulge in unhealthy foods, whether we are addicted to them or not, our bodies know it. And, whether it's a subconscious occurrence or not, we often punish ourselves. We know that we are doing something wrong. We feel upset about it and dissatisfied, even if we are processing it in the moment.

Processed foods are also high in artificial colorings that have been proven to be highly carcinogenic. When we are eating foods that have fixed coloring in it, we are essentially

swallowing
dye. Would you want to eat hair dye? Not really. But these types of chemicals are what are used in your food. They stay in your body and do not come out. They dye your organs on the inside. They are highly dangerous and can lead to cancer.

There also full of preservatives. Processed food stays on the

shelf
for a very long time. Longer than is healthy and normal. Any

typical bottle of milk would not last for months on end at a time. It would curdle and spoil. The same as with cheeses, and the same as with other foods that you find on the shelves that have long shelf lives.

Shelf lives are important for companies to establish because

they
are able to make more money if their food is able to stay on the shelf longer. They will do whatever it takes, whether it is healthier not to the human body, to ensure that they are making the most money possible.

Preservatives often include unhealthy and unnatural chemicals and excessive amounts of salt. Neither of which are good for the body at all. Processed foods can lead to issues with the heart, and hypertension, because of the excessive amount of salt present in these foods. High blood pressure is a common occurrence among people who survive off of processed foods, and obesity and heart attacks are some of the number one killer's in North America.

This has absolutely everything to do with the standard American diet. The sad part about it is that even if you know it is unhealthy,
the chemicals and high sugar and fat content make these processed foods extremely addicting.

The body begins to crave them, and it can be almost as dangerous as a drug addiction. When you are addicted to a food that is neither nourishing nor healthy, it can have long-term consequences on your health and development.

Another way that processed foods contribute to obesity is because we digest them far too quickly compared to foods that are rich in healthy dietary fiber. If we are digesting these foods quickly and they are not filling us up because we are not receiving the fiber that provides us with the full feeling, we are not even burning the same amount of energy as we would to digest healthy foods.

This means that we eat more and digest less, leading to fast and rapid weight gain. The calories present in your body are much higher when you are on a diet of processed foods. You burn far more calories when you are eating healthy, whole foods that are rich in dietary fibers.

Unfortunately, this means that people who live and subsist on a diet of processed foods are ultimately going to gain weight whether they want to or not. And they will not provide you with the same amount of energy because they are not nourishing. They are likely to leave you tired and sluggish, and feeling far

too
full because you eat a lot more of these unhealthy, sugar filled foods without feeling content or satiated.
Processed food is not metabolized properly in our bodies. They are quickly turned to fat. Not only that, but they are high in fat. They are often full of hidden fat and sugars. Vegetable oil is one of the primary ingredients in many of these processed meals,

along with things such as high fructose corn syrup, which is a huge culprit in weight gain.

If every processed food on the shelves contained high fructose corn syrup, and most of them do, it is no wonder that North America is facing the worst obesity epidemic in the world

history.
Hydrogenated oils are highly unhealthy because they do not break down.

They remain in your body and become merged with the fat cells. These oils make fat far more difficult to burn off. They are harder to get rid of, and that type of stubborn fat can lead to obesity very quickly. The ingredients in processed foods lack most of the nutritional value that humans need in order to function at their highest potential. We need the fibers and the vitamins and minerals that are present in real food before we can truly thrive.

If you find that processed foods can't be entirely avoided, they should at least be eaten in moderation. They are dangerous. They can make us feel sluggish, irritable, and unhappy overall.

Our dispositions can go from positive to negative when we go from a healthy diet and ultimately find ourselves consumed with nothing but processed foods that are too sugary, too fatty, and to unhealthy.

Our bodies crave nutrition. The easiest and most beneficial thing you can do for yourself is to provide your body with that nutrition. It can be hard to get used to changing of routines such as subsisting off of processed foods, and it can be very frustrating at times.

You have to spend a lot more time in the kitchen cooking and taking your health and your meals into consideration. But ultimately, eating processed foods is something that can kill you and cut you off from yourself. You are actually consuming toxins and avoiding the foods that can act as antioxidants that will provide you with a chance to get rid of the waste that you are putting into your body.

Processed foods are the same as junk foods. They are no different. They are healthier seeming junk foods. They are snacks in disguise. In order to become healthy and to actually feel healthy, avoiding processed foods at all costs is the first and most effective step that you can take. Don't let yourself be fooled by packaging that claims these foods are healthy.

They are saturated and fat and sugar and salt, and lacking in anything that gives your body nourishment. Do everything you can to change your habit of relying on processed foods. Eating healthy is easy and possible if you set your mind to it.

Just remember the strategy of walking around the grocery store to pick up the fresh produce and meat as opposed to walking through the aisles that are full of dangerous and alluring packaging that is hiding the dangers of the processed food within.

CHAPTER 10: BRINGING IT ALL TOGETHER WITH MEAL PLANNING

Meal planning can be one of the single most important aspects of developing a healthy lifestyle. When we are unable to visualize the future of our eating, it can be very easy to succumb to the temptations of unhealthy foods that we have become addicted to. Especially if it is our habit to eat them rather than eating the foods that will nourish us.

Meal planning is quite an endeavor. It can be somewhat intimidating, especially to somebody who suffers with organization. If you find yourself having a hard time with meal planning, don't fret. There are many ways that you can begin to delve into meal planning that are fun and easy, whether you struggle with creativity in the kitchen or not.

There are many meal planning kits that you can buy. Many of them have the option of ordering boxes full of fresh foods to cook with and include recipes that you can use. This can be very helpful if you are not used to cooking, which is often the case.

Especially when poor eating habits and a busy work schedule make it seem difficult to carve out the time necessary in order to make full, nourishing meals. The first step in meal planning is research. If you are going to get yourself healthy, you have to look at your options.

Researching recipes is the best first place to start. Accumulating a binder full of healthy foods that you want to try out can be both fun and educational. It will open your mind to several food possibilities you may have otherwise scoffed at as too difficult for you to prepare, or maybe teach you things you had never known before.

Recipes can be very mind-opening. Especially when you are interested in making new discoveries. Cooking can be a hard habit to get into, but once you begin to master it, you will be surprised by just how much freedom you can find in putting a meal together for yourself that is both health-conscious and delicious!

Look at recipe books and magazines and get an accumulation of recipes that you want to try. Start with the things that look the most delicious and nourishing, and if you are a novice in the kitchen, you may also want to look to the things that seem the most simple.

Next, you should keep your recipes organized in a simple way that is easy to navigate. If you find yourself overwhelmed by a lack of organization, it will make meal planning that much more difficult.

When you are beginning a new habit, you want to make sure that you are doing everything as simply as possible. Too much change at once can be demanding on your system, and you should always try to implement small, easy changes until they have become a new habit.

Make sure that they are easily accessible, so that when you want to begin preparing your meal you can do so easily. If you are using a binder, you may want to consider laminating the pages or using plastic sleeves, so that if you are using it in the kitchen, they are not affected by water or other food contamination.

When you organize your recipes, it would help to put them in order of breakfast meals, lunch meals, dinner meals, and snacks. This will help you to reference the proper recipes more easily once you begin to start cooking. If you like, you could even organize your binder by day of the week, and have your meals planned out for every day and printed out in the binder that way.

There are many ways you could organize your recipes. Do what seems to make the most sense to you intuitively. Don't force yourself to adhere to a type of organization that doesn't work for you. Instead, make sure that you are doing what works best for you in your own life.

Make sure that you are taking the time to regularly seek out new recipes that stand out to you to keep your creative juices flowing and your kitchen exciting. There are many types of recipes you can try, and the more you attempt, the more interesting going on a journey of healthy eating can be!

Next, you should explore software such as Excel on Microsoft Office that will help you to organize your meal planning. On Excel you will find a plethora of templates you can choose from to help yourself plan out your meals by the day, time, and week. This can be a hugely valuable resource!

If you would prefer not to use excel, there are also apps you could download on your phone or tablet or another device to help you to utilize your time and resources better.

You can even go the old fashioned route and buy a notebook that is specially designed toward planning meals. This is an important step in making sure your meals are organized and easily accessible.

Having a meal plan is extremely helpful when it comes to embarking upon a journey of healthy eating. Creating good habits takes time and patience, and it is inevitable that you will slip somewhere along the way.

But that doesn't mean that you have to stay stuck on the ground! Actually, it just means that you are going to have to get back up and keep trying, because giving up is far easier than sticking to your plans.

One thing that can really help when it comes to meal planning is sticking with the theme. For example, a lot of people have specific themes like taco Tuesday or another day that is

assigned
for a specific type of meal. If you think that would help you to stay on track, feel free to imitate that type of meal planning. It is done for a reason, because it works and it helps to keep things simple and streamlined.

It can be very annoying to find yourself stuck doing a lot of planning and preparation every single week or month, so if you want to keep things easy, that can be a good way to do it. You could have a theme for biweekly meals, such as taco Tuesday one night and maybe rice and vegetables Tuesday the next and alternate between them. There is no wrong way to plan your meals. What you have to make sure you do is to observe follow through.

Without follow-through, everything else becomes redundant and difficult. Something that can truly help you to succeed at meal planning is accountability. If you let somebody who knows you and cares about you know that you are attempting to plan your meals, ask them if they would be willing to help you to stick to your routine.

They can help you by asking questions about how things are going and whether or not you are staying on track. They may also choose to encourage you and cheer you on through your endeavors.

However they choose to support you, they can be very rewarding for both of you. If they are a positive and supportive person, it can be great to know that you have people rallied in your corner who truly want you to succeed. Just make sure that you are weeding out toxic people who bring you down by turning the attention onto themselves or by making you feel as if it will be difficult for you to accomplish your goals.

Sure, constructive feedback can be incredibly useful, but if you are not seeking constructive feedback, it can at times be toxic. Make sure you understand the difference between a toxic person masquerading as a supportive person and a supportive person who truly wants to see you thrive.

Another way to take accountability is by taking personal accountability. Personal accountability can be achieved through journaling and self affirmations. Talking to yourself about your goals, what do you do it internally or out loud, can be a good way to help you to stay focused and ask yourself whether or not you are doing the things that you hope to accomplish.

If you find that you are not, instead of beating yourself up about it, consider your obstacles and move on as you begin to uncover them. The only way you will ever be a failure is if you do not try. If you try, everything will ultimately fall into place because you are making an effort and creating positive changes in your life.

Journaling is useful for many reasons. They can help you to

write
down what you have eaten and when and how much. This will give you a good idea of what you can realistically expect from yourself. The things that you are unhappy with, you should address and take note of. But instead of being angry at yourself for not being a trickle right away, remember that it is a process and you need to go slowly.

Instead of implementing an entire change in routine and planning out every meal for the next month when you have never done it before, instead, start slow by easing into one or two meals a week, and then gradually adding in the rest as you feel comfortable with the process.
Make it something that does not shock your system. Gradual change is the most lasting. And journaling about your experiences will help you to uncover your innermost thoughts about the process and things that you might not even realize were holding you back.

You will begin to sense patterns in your behavior and possibly predict when you might find yourself tempted to get off track and why. If you are able to identify these trigger points, it will be easier to avoid them in the future.

Meal planning can be a very fun and exciting endeavor. Even if you aren't the type who enjoys that type of organization, it can be very rewarding to think about exactly what you are going to be putting in your body and take the steps necessary in actually doing so. Everybody deserves a chance to become the

healthiest
and most healthy version of themselves possible, and with meal planning and a healthy dose of self-esteem, you will be well on your way to a lifestyle of healthy eating.

CONCLUSION

Healthy eating is something that can be very difficult to begin doing, especially if you were not able to develop healthy eating habits from a young age. However, it is not impossible to become a more health conscious and proactive person.

Fortunately, every single day that we wake up living and breathing is a day that we can begin to better ourselves and move forward in our lives.

Becoming the best version of ourselves can seem intimidating at first, but once you start to realize that every choice you make has an impact on your life, whether positive or negative, then it becomes a lot easier to see the course of our actions before they come back to haunt us. Poor eating habits are definitely choices that will come back to haunt us.

If we are not careful, we will begin to develop health problems later in life because we were not conscientious of what we put into our bodies when we were younger. Healthy eating and exercise is the only way to create a healthy and happy body and mind.

We become stir crazy and restless when we stay stuck in our homes all day eating nothing but sugar and fat laden processed foods and sitting around watching TV without exercising. The standard American diet is dangerous, and it is costing people their lives. Don't let yourself become one of those people.

Instead, make the choices that you need to make in order to truly better yourself and become the best version of yourself possible. Make choices that will make your family proud and will provide them with your presence in their lives for years to come.

When we are not taking care of ourselves, this is actually very selfish. There are people around us who care deeply for the people that we are and the value that we bring to their lives, whether we realize it or not. Everybody deserves a chance to take their future into their own hands and create positive changes that will benefit them for years to come.

Healthy eating is just one of many ways that you can begin to better yourself and prepare your mind and body for the future. If you want to be independent and active for as long as possible without costing yourself thousands upon thousands of dollars in medical bills and other expenses, then healthy eating is something that you should begin sooner rather than later.

If not, it is bound to become a drain on your life, both materially and physically. By reading this book and utilizing the information within it, you are now more prepared for taking the first step toward a healthy lifestyle.

Planning your meals and becoming more aware of why it is important to make healthy food choices will drastically improve your quality of life now and for years to come. All you have to do is stick with it, and you will begin to see the positive health effects of healthy eating right away! All you have to do is try. You can do this!

www.ingramcontent.com/pod-product-compliance
Lightning Source LLC
Chambersburg PA
CBHW081604250726
48653CB00009B/3553